# RODNEY DANGERFIELD

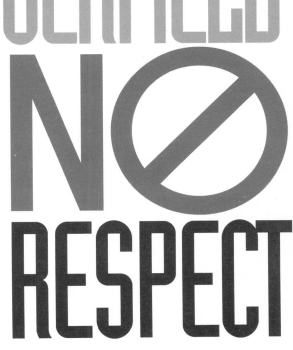

NO RESPECT

Rodney Dangerfield

Illustrated by Bill & Eric Teitlebaum

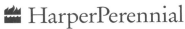

**HarperPerennial**
*A Division of* HarperCollins*Publishers*

HarperCollins books may be purchased for educational, business, or sales promotional use. For information please write: Special Markets Department, HarperCollins Publishers, Inc., 10 East 53rd Street, New York, NY 10022.

FIRST EDITION

*Designed by William Delorme*

ISBN 0-06-095117-6

95 96 97 98 99 ❖/HC 10 9 8 7 6 5 4 3 2

I TELL YA, with me nothing works out. I always get stuck. That's how I got my name, RODNEY DANGERFIELD.

When I went into show business I saw an ad in the paper. It said: "Improve Your Personality..." So I went to see the man.

He told me my personality was okay, but my name was my problem.

I said to him, "My name? How could a name be a problem? Even William Shakespeare said, 'What's in a name?'"

He said, "Who?"

I said, "William Shakespeare."

He said, "Look, do you want to listen to me, or do you want to listen to your friends?"

I said to him, "I don't understand. Is it good to change your name?"

He said, "Of course. I always keep changing my name. In fact, right now I can give you a very good deal. I can give you a new name for five hundred dollars."

I said, "Five hundred dollars! That's a lot of money!"

He said, "It's a great name. It's a name, once people hear it, they'll start saying it."

I said, "What's the name?"

He said, "Rodney Dangerfield."

I said, "RODNEY DANGERFIELD?"

He said, "See, you just heard it, and you're starting to say it! Listen to me, take the name."

I said, "Wait a minute. Suppose I take the name and I don't like it. Can I bring it back?"

He said, "Of course. All I ask is one thing. While you're using the name, don't give it a bad name."

So I decided to call myself Rodney Dangerfield. As soon as I got home, I thought to myself, I made a mistake. I called the guy up. I said, "Look, I want my money back. This is Rodney Dangerfield."

He said, "Who?"

I said, "Dangerfield. Don't you remember?"

He said, "Oh, yeah, Shakespeare's friend."

I said, "Look, I don't want the name."

He said, "Don't be foolish. Try it for two weeks. I guarantee you'll like it."

I tried the name for two weeks, I still didn't like it. I went to bring it back. I couldn't find the guy.

He changed his name!

*Rodney Dangerfield*

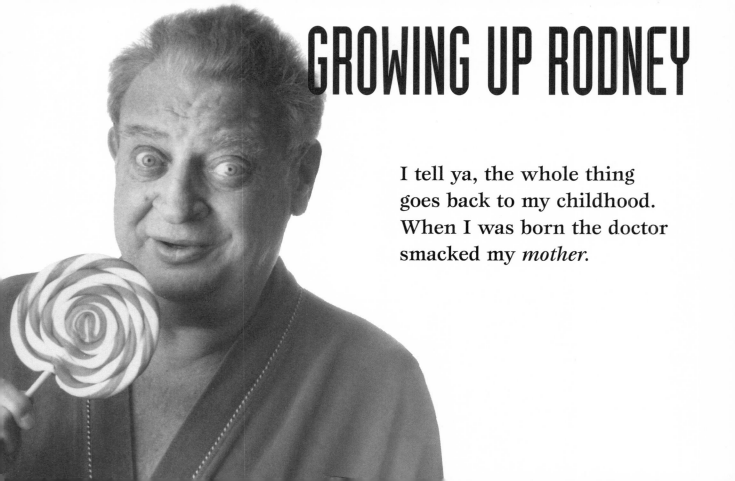

# GROWING UP RODNEY

I tell ya, the whole thing goes back to my childhood. When I was born the doctor smacked my *mother*.

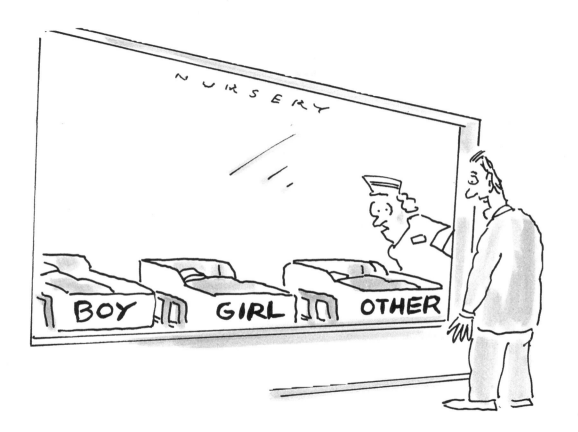

5

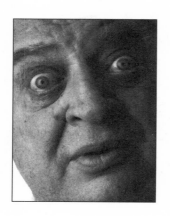

What a childhood....
I was breast-fed by my *father*.

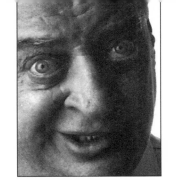

Why, when I was born, the doctor
told my mother, "I did all I could do,
but he pulled through anyway."

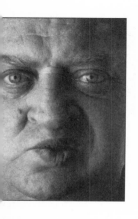

When I was born I got no respect.
After the doctor smacked me,
the *nurses* got in a few.

For my birthday, my ole man
showed me a picture of a cake....
I sat there all day trying
to blow out the candles.

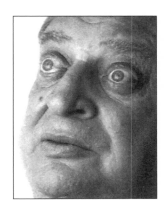

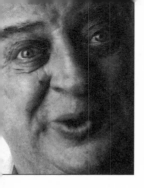

Until I was six years old
I thought Alpo was baby food.

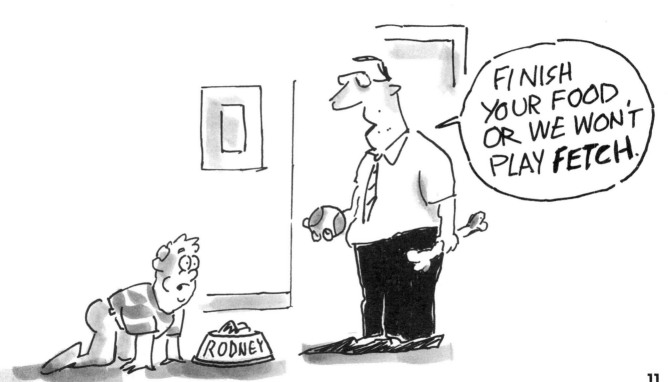

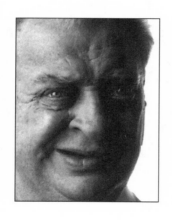

My ole man told me never
to take candy from a stranger...
unless he offered me a ride.

What a childhood I had.
When I was kidnapped, they sent
back a piece of my finger....
My ole man said he wanted more proof.

I remember the note they sent.
"We want $5,000, or you'll
see your son again."

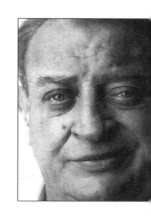

I was an ugly kid, too. Every time my ole man wanted sex, my mother showed him my picture.

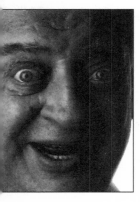

Why, I was so ugly, they made *me* the poster boy for Birth Control.

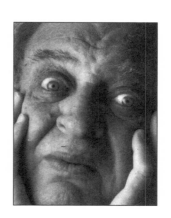

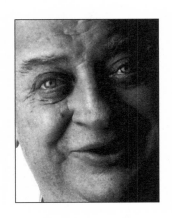

I had plenty of pimples, too.  I fell asleep in the library.... I woke up and a blind man was reading my face.

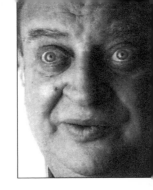

In the park I had no friends.
I remember the seesaw.... I had to
keep running from one end to the other.

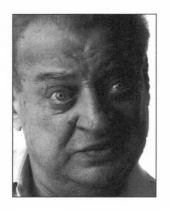

When I played in the sandbox,
the cat kept covering me up all the time.

When I was a kid, I got no respect at all....
Why, my yo-yo, it never came back.

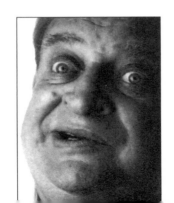

I asked my ole man if I could
go ice-skating on the lake.
He told me to wait till it gets warmer.

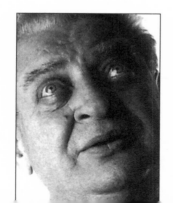

I remember one day, I told
my ole man, "I'm sick and tired
of running around in circles."
He had nailed down my other foot.

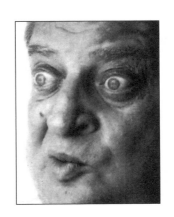

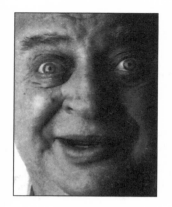

Once I stuck my head out the window
and got arrested for mooning.

When I was a kid it was different.
I had it rough.... My ole man kept
taking me to the zoo.... I found out
he was trying to make a trade.

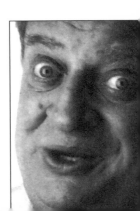

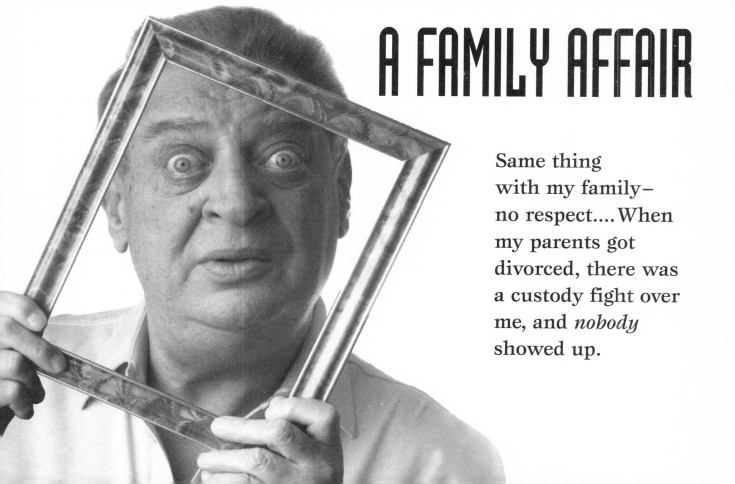

# A FAMILY AFFAIR

Same thing with my family– no respect.... When my parents got divorced, there was a custody fight over me, and *nobody* showed up.

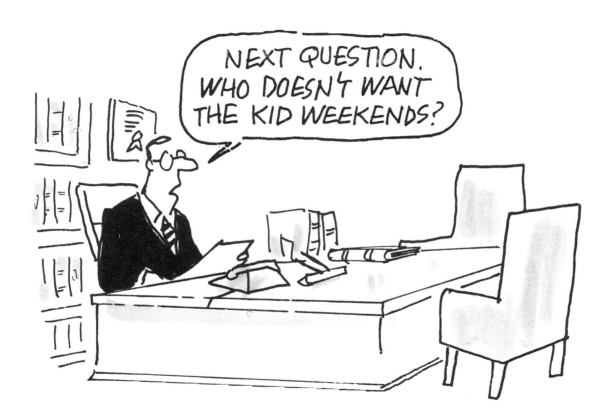

25

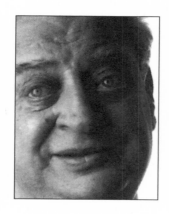

I looked up my family tree...
two dogs were using it.

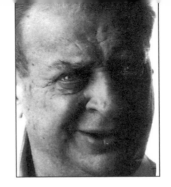

What a family. My ole man
told me to start at the bottom....
He was teaching me how to swim.

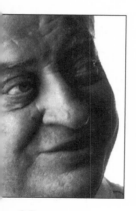

I didn't get respect from anyone.
My twin brother forgot my birthday.

Why, my uncle's dying wish,
he wanted me on his lap....
He was in the electric chair.

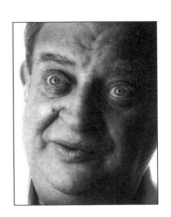

# A FAMILY AFFAIR

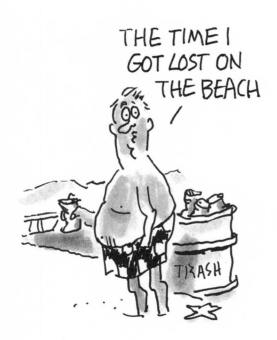

THE TIME I GOT LOST ON THE BEACH

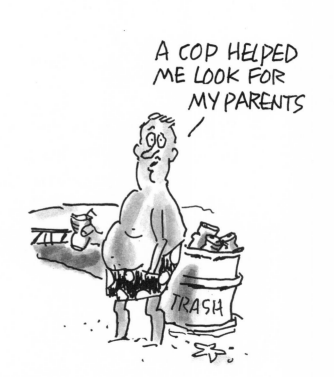

A COP HELPED ME LOOK FOR MY PARENTS

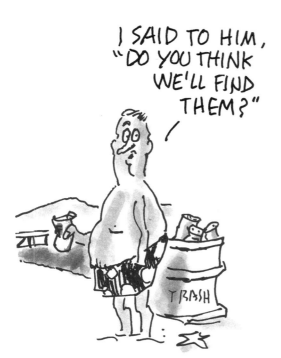

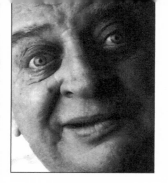

My ole man gave the lifeguard $5 to keep an eye *off* me.

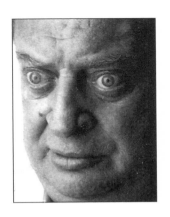

When my ole man took me hunting,
that was a beauty.... On the way home
he tied me to the fender and put
the *deer* in the car.

My ole man was dumb, too.... He worked
in a bank— they caught him stealing pens.

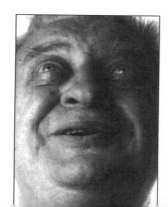

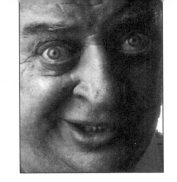

I tell ya, he was *dumb*. He wouldn't
buy Christmas Seals...he said he
wouldn't know what to feed them.

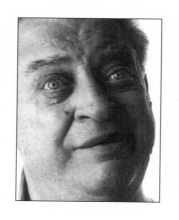

My ole man...one time he picked
a guy's pocket on an airplane
and tried to make a run for it.

Oh, he was strict.... He allowed no drinking in the house. I had two brothers who died of thirst.

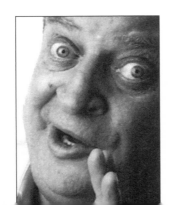

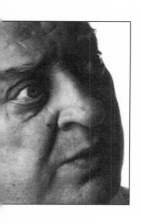

My ole man still carries around the picture of the kid who came with his wallet.

When we used to play catch,
he dropped me.

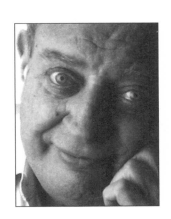

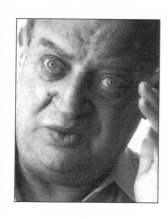

My mother never breast-fed me....
She told me she liked me as a friend.

She had morning sickness *after* I was born.

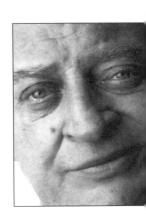

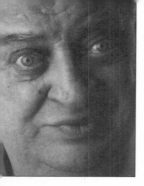

We were poor, too.... If I wasn't a boy, I would have had *nothing* to play with.

Easter! They gave me
chocolate bunnies made of Ex-Lax.

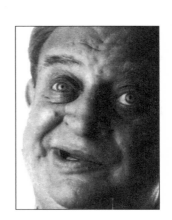

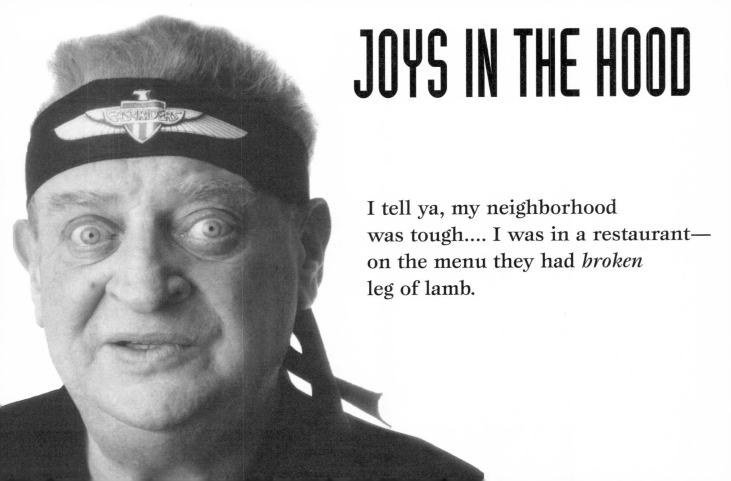

# JOYS IN THE HOOD

I tell ya, my neighborhood
was tough.... I was in a restaurant—
on the menu they had *broken*
leg of lamb.

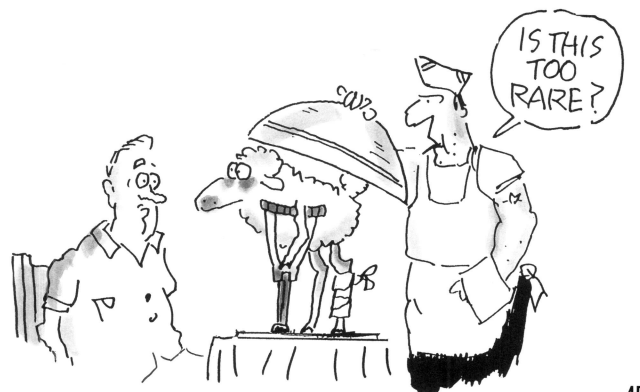

45

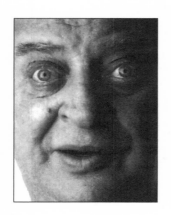

One time a guy pulled a knife
on me.... I could tell it wasn't
a professional job; it had butter on it.

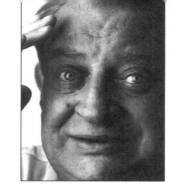

What a neighborhood....
I had it tough....
I bought a water bed, there was
a guy at the bottom of it.

47

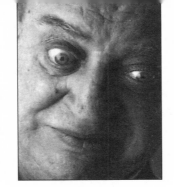

Nothin' but crime…. Every time I closed the window, I hit somebody's hands.

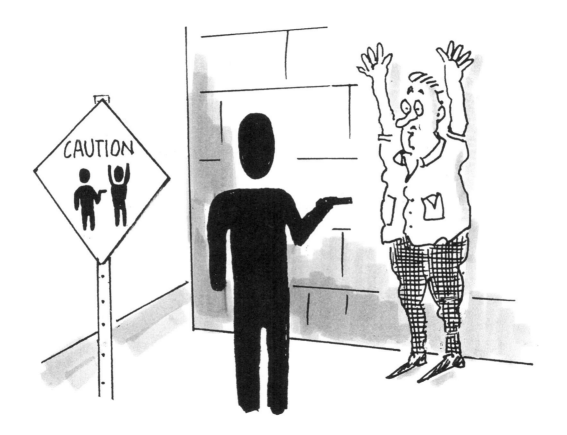

49

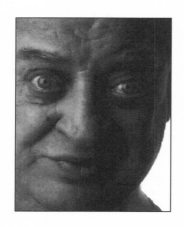

Last week on my block they raffled off a police car...with two cops still in it.

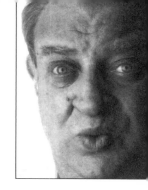

In the police station the front door has a *peephole*.

I knew I was in trouble when I rented the apartment. The ad in the paper said, "Short run to subway."

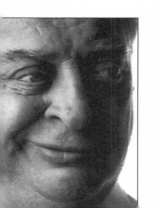

It's a tough neighborhood.
There was a knock on my door.
I figured I'd play it safe
and open the peephole....
A guy reached in and
grabbed me—with *both* hands.

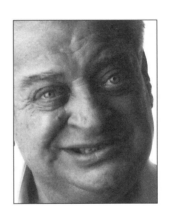

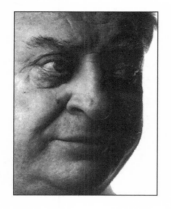

I don't get no respect from anyone.
The time I wanted to jump off the roof,
a priest came up to talk to me.
He said, "On your mark."

I was in a bar. They told me
to get out...they wanted to start
the happy hour.

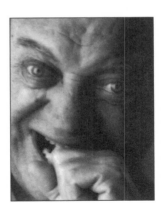

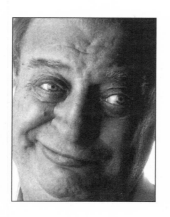

In my neighborhood I got no respect....
Halloween! Parents sent their kids out
looking like *me*.

Last year a kid tried to rip my face off.

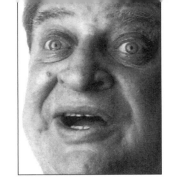

I tell ya, I can't take it anymore....
I bought a funeral plot. The guy said,
"There goes the neighborhood."

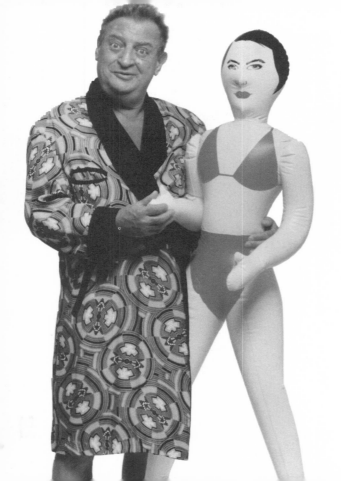

# KISS & TELL: THE DATING YEARS

With girls I never had any luck. I made love to an inflatable girl...now I've got an inflatable guy looking for me.

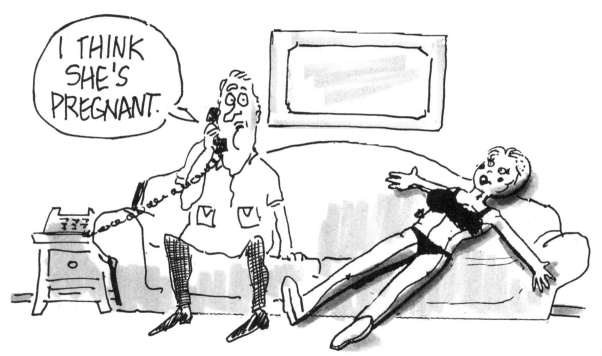

59

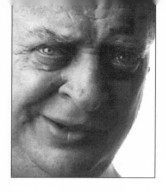

# KISS & TELL: THE DATING YEARS

With girls I don't get no respect.
I was making love to one girl,
she started to cry. I said to her,
"You'll hate yourself in the morning."
She said, "No, I hate myself *now*."

One time I had a blind date.
I waited two hours on the corner.
A girl walked by.
I said, "Are you Louise?"
She said, "Are you Rodney?"
I said, "Yeah."
She said, "I'm not Louise."

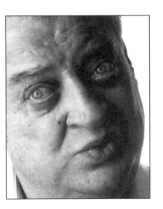

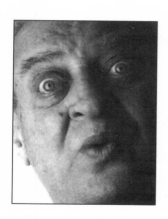

I had a blind date — she was a wild girl....
She made French toast and her tongue
got caught in the toaster.

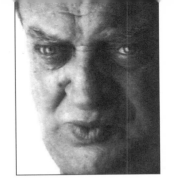

Blind dates never work out.
I always get losers....
One girl showed up, she had
pigtails under her *arms*.

With me, nothin' works out.
I bought a book, <u>100 Ways to Make Love</u>.... I ended up in traction... there was a misprint.

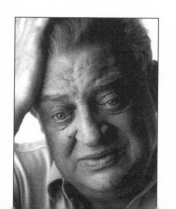

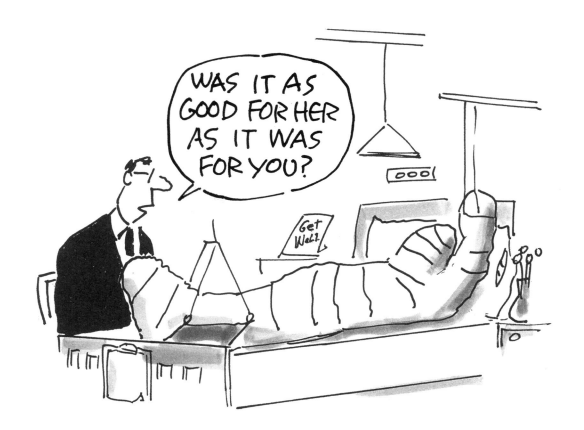

65

# KISS & TELL: THE DATING YEARS

I tell ya, girls never went for me....
I took out a belly dancer,
she told me I turned her stomach.

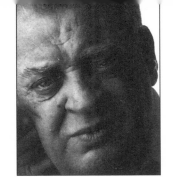

A hooker once told me she had a headache.

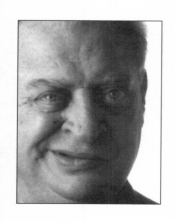

I went to a discount massage parlor...
it was self-service.

My big thrill was self-inflicted hickies.

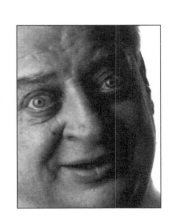

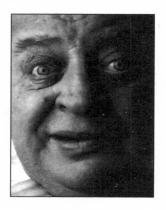

# KISS & TELL: THE DATING YEARS

I love two girls at once.... If I fall asleep, they got each other to talk to.

When it comes to sex, I want
a good girl, a girl who's never
played around.... I figure she's due.

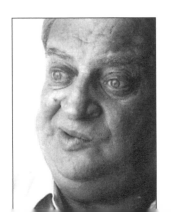

If it wasn't for pickpockets,
I'd have no sex life at all.

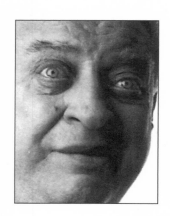

I *know* I'm a bad lover....
I caught a peeping Tom booing me.

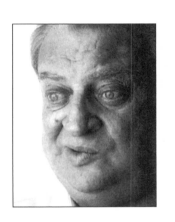

This girl was ugly.  She went to
a plastic surgeon.... He added a tail.

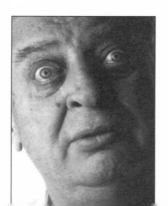

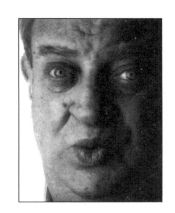

When she walked into a room
*mice* jumped on chairs.

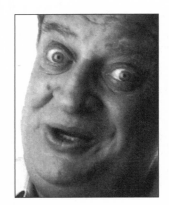

I tell ya, this girl was ugly.
She looked like she came in second
in a hatchet fight.

They used her in prison
to cure sex offenders.

I took her to a dog show and she won.

The last time I saw a mouth like that
it had a hook in it.

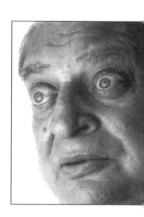

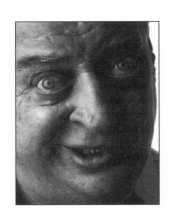

I went out with a girl. Boy, was she fat.... She got on a scale and a card came out saying, "One at a time."

Her *bathtub* had stretch marks.

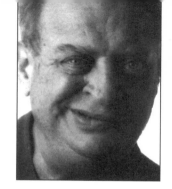

Her belly button made an echo.

Her bikini was made out of two sheets.

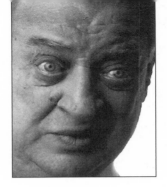

# KISS & TELL: THE DATING YEARS

One day, I hit her with my car.
When she asked why I didn't
go around her, I told her,
"I didn't have enough gas."

Fat. You kidding!
When she went swimming
she left a ring around the lake.

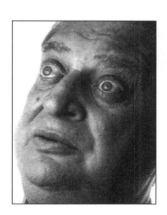

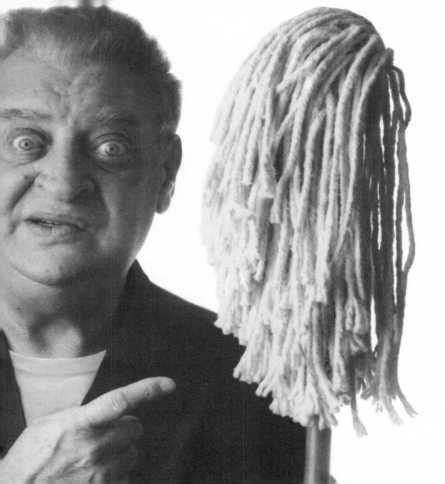

# BALL & CHAIN: MRS. RODNEY

I tell ya, with my wife, life isn't easy. Last night she told me to take out the garbage. I told her, "You cooked it, *you* take it out."

83

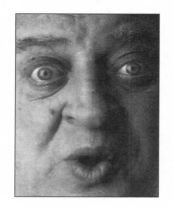

# BALL & CHAIN: MRS. RODNEY

She can't cook at all. When we have
a picnic I bring along Tums for the ants.

I've got the only dog that begs
for Alka-Seltzer.

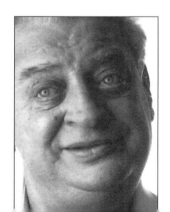

I leave dental floss in the kitchen
and watch the roaches hang themselves.

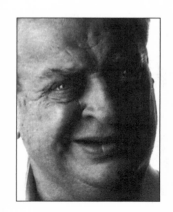

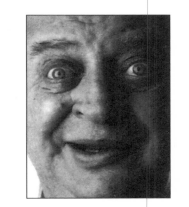

You've heard of, "Come and get it."
In my house it's, "Try and *eat* it."

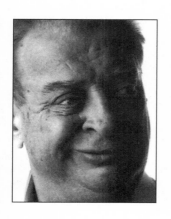

Last night my wife told me to take out the garbage.  I told her I already took out the garbage.... Then she told me to go out and keep an eye on it.

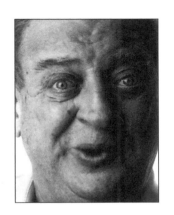

I told my wife when I die,
I want to be cremated....
She's planning a barbeque.

# BALL & CHAIN: MRS. RODNEY

And the way she drives, that's something....
She has a pair of shoes over the dashboard...
they belong to the last guy she hit.

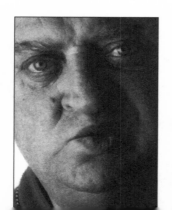

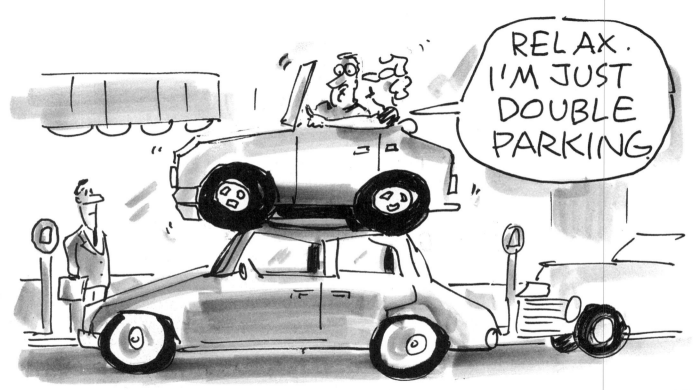

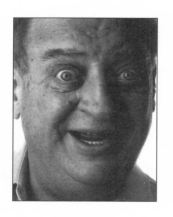

Last week she hit a deer...
it was in the zoo.

One time a guy stole the car.
I asked my wife if she saw
what the guy looked like....
She said, "No, but I got the
license plate number."

My wife signed me up
for the Bridge Club....
I jump off next Tuesday.

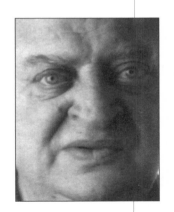

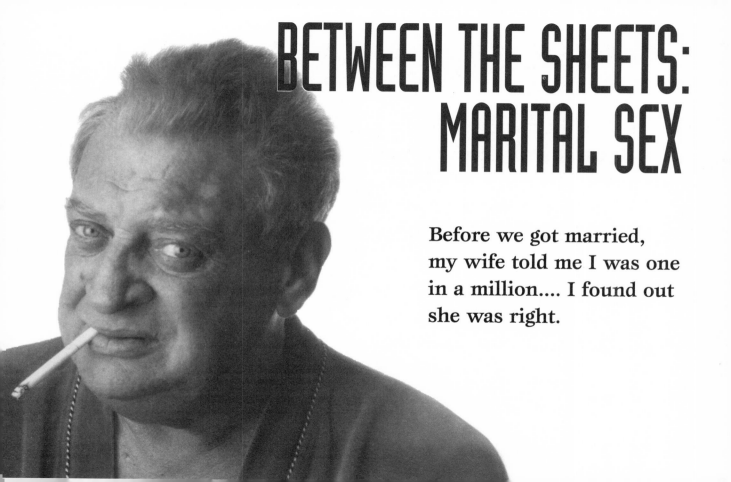

# BETWEEN THE SHEETS: MARITAL SEX

Before we got married, my wife told me I was one in a million.... I found out she was right.

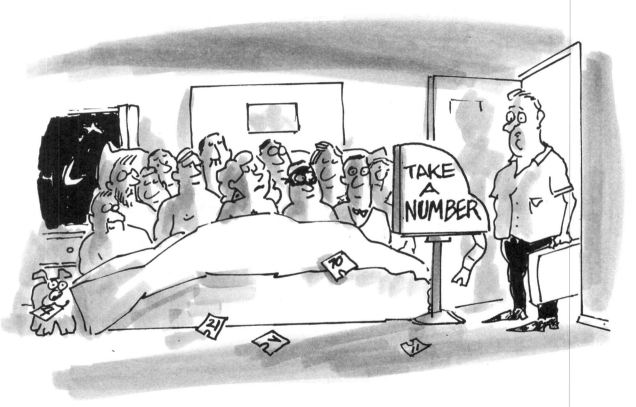

# BETWEEN THE SHEETS: MARITAL SEX

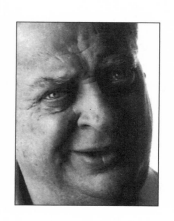

My wife drives me nuts.
She was afraid of the dark....
She saw me naked...
now she's afraid of the *light*.

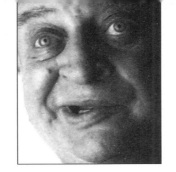

I asked her if she enjoys a cigarette after sex. She said, "No. One drag is enough."

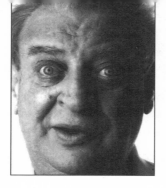

# BETWEEN THE SHEETS: MARITAL SEX

My wife.... All we do is fight
about money and sex....
I mean, she *charges* me too much.

With my wife nothin' comes easy....
When I want sex she leaves the room
to give me privacy.

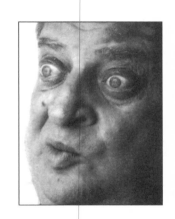

# BETWEEN THE SHEETS: MARITAL SEX

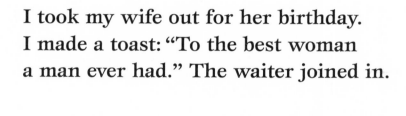

I took my wife out for her birthday.
I made a toast: "To the best woman
a man ever had." The waiter joined in.

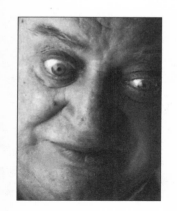

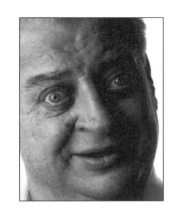

My wife told me she wanted sex
in the backseat of a car....
I drove her and that guy around all night.

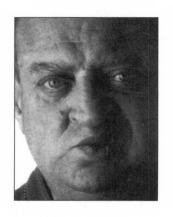

I tell ya, when my wife has sex
with me, there's always a reason....
Last night she used me to time an egg.

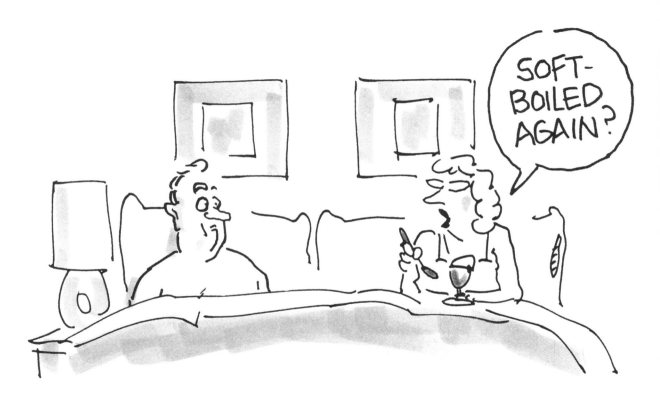

The other night she was sleeping.
I heard her saying sexy things....
I looked up, she was on the phone.

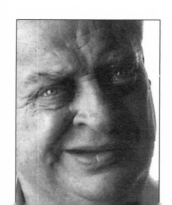

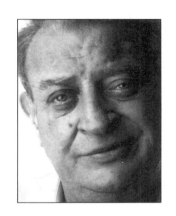

Last night my wife met me
at the front door. She was wearing
a sexy negligee.... The only trouble
was, she was coming home.

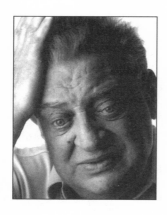

# BETWEEN THE SHEETS: MARITAL SEX

With her I got no sex life....
She keeps trying to mate the dog
and tells *me* to get fixed.

I asked a cab driver, "Where can I get some action?" He took me to my house.

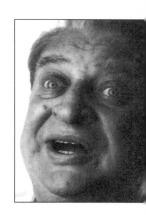

During sex, my wife likes to talk to me....
The other night she called me from a motel.

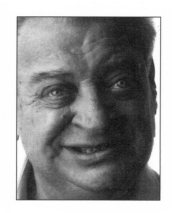

108

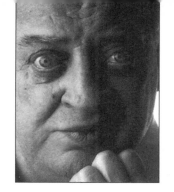

One night I figured I'd let her make
the first move.... She went to Florida.

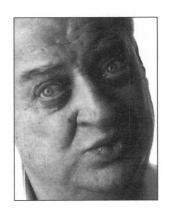

I tell ya, with me, nothing works out.
My marriage is on the rocks....
My wife broke up with her boyfriend.

I tell ya, with me, nothing comes easy....
This morning I did my push-ups
in the nude.... I didn't see the mousetrap.

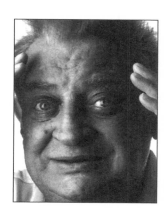

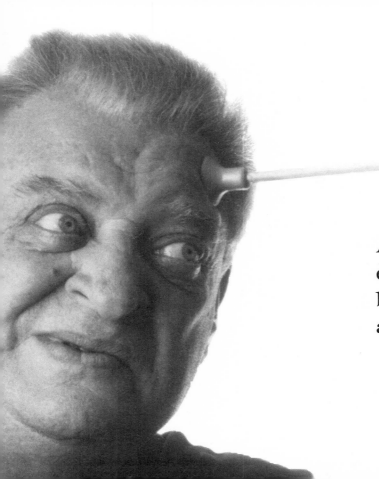

# PRIDE & JOY

And my kid, he don't help either.... I told him all about the birds and the bees.... He went out and knocked up a sparrow.

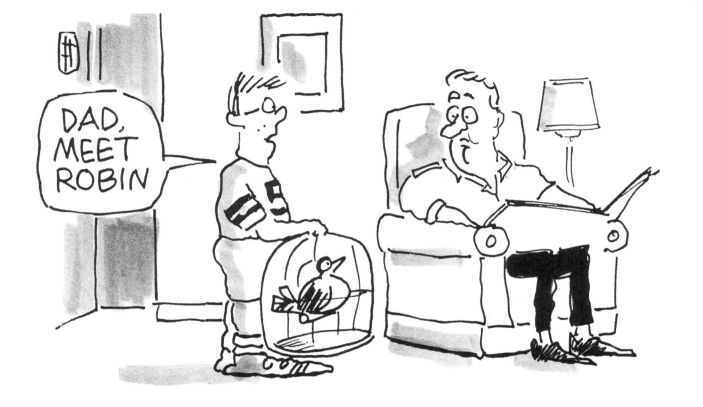

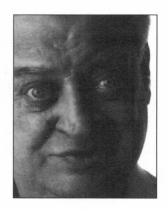

I told my kid, "Someday you'll
have children of your own...."
He said, "So will you."

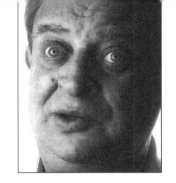

For Christmas I gave my kid
a BB gun. He gave me a sweatshirt
with a bull's-eye in the back.

My kid is mean. He Scotch-tapes worms to the sidewalk and then watches the birds get hernias.

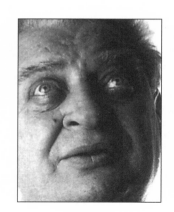

He wants to be a prison warden
when he grows up, so he can
put thumbtacks on the electric chair.

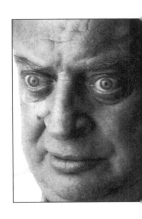

# PRIDE & JOY

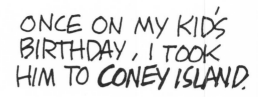

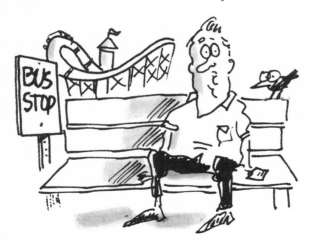

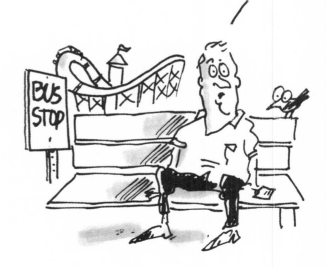

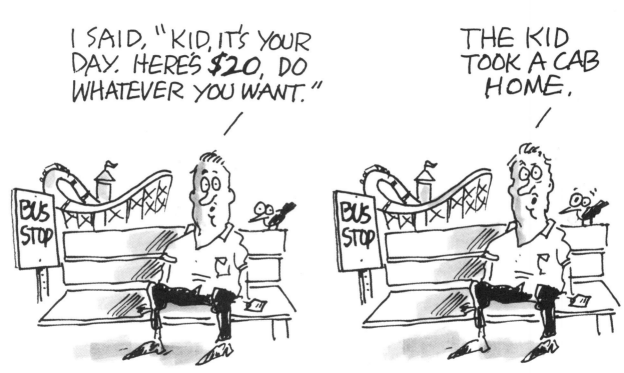

119

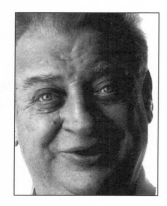

I tell ya, nothin' goes right.
Last week I found a guy's wallet...
inside was a picture of my two kids.

I tell ya, with my kid,
I don't get no respect.
I told him, "You're young,
you don't have it upstairs."
He told me, "You're old,
you don't have it *downstairs*."

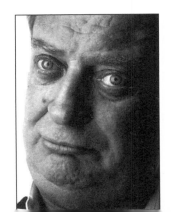

My daughter's no bargain, either.
In public school she was voted
most likely to conceive.

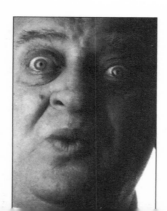

She flunked her driver's test....
She couldn't get used to the *front* seat.

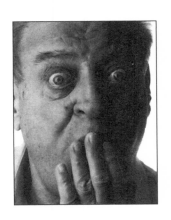

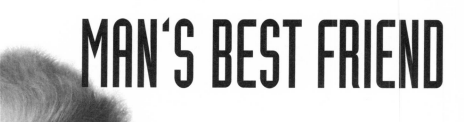

# MAN'S BEST FRIEND

My dog, that's another one. He keeps barking at the front door.... He don't want to go out.... He wants *me* to leave.

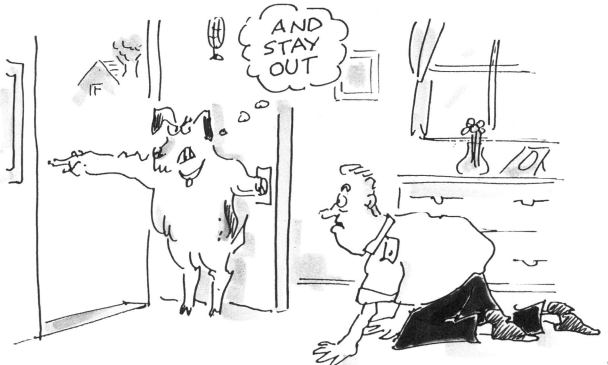

125

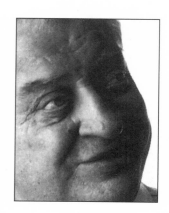

What a dog I've got....
His favorite bone is my arm.

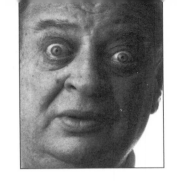

And he's lazy, too....
He don't chase cars....
He sits on the curb and
takes down license plate numbers.

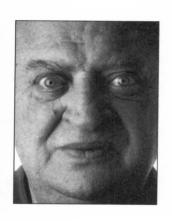

I tell ya, the dog drives me nuts.
Last night he went on the paper
four times...three times
while I was reading it.

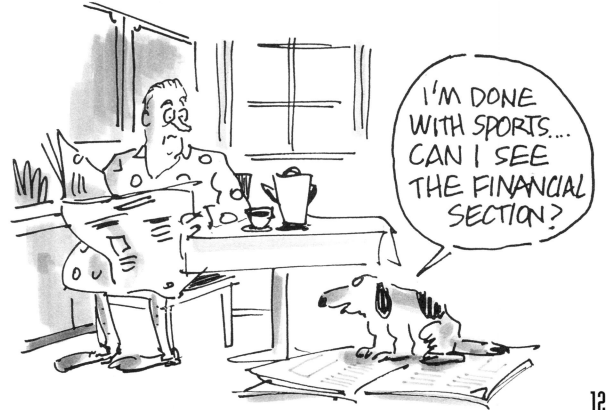

129

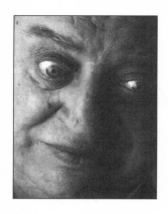

# MAN'S BEST FRIEND

I got no sex life.... My dog keeps watching me in the bedroom.... He wants to learn how to beg.

He taught my wife how to roll over and play dead.

And my wife, she don't help either....
She kisses the dog on the lips,
and she won't drink from *my* glass.

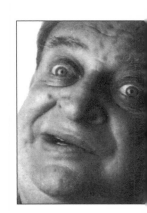

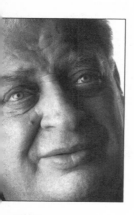

I tell ya, my dog makes me feel
like I'm dirty.... He jumps on the bed
and smells it for a half hour
before he lays down on it.

I call my dog Egypt....
Every room, he leaves a pyramid.

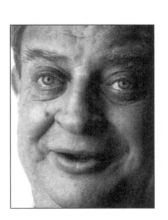

Nothing works out. I donated to a sperm bank....
Now I'm the father of three puppies.

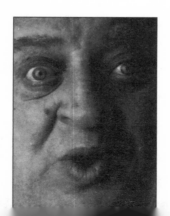

134

My dog found out we look alike....
He killed himself.

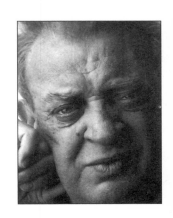

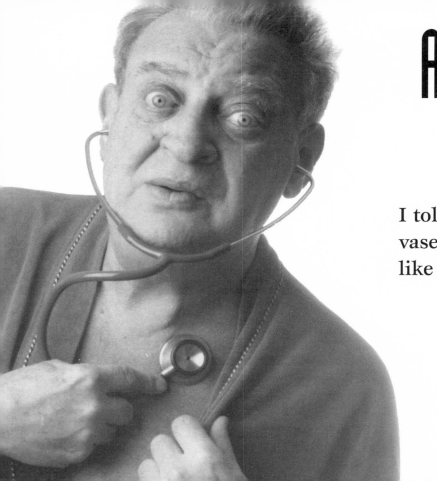

# ACHES & PAINS

I told my doctor I want a
vasectomy. He said with a face
like mine, I don't need one.

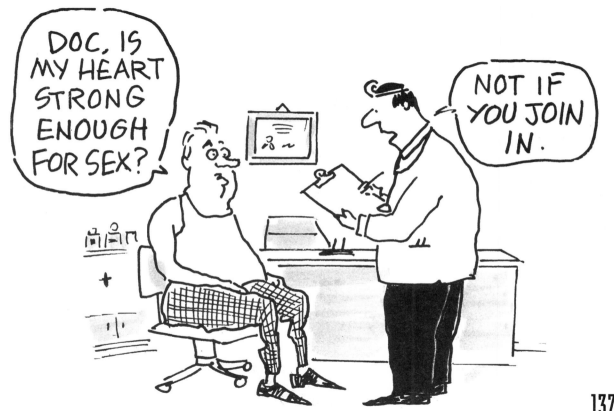

137

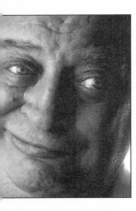

I tried group sex....
That didn't work out either....
I don't know who to thank.

You know my doctor — Dr. Vinny Boombatz.
I told him I swallowed a bottle of
sleeping pills. He told me to have
a few drinks and get some rest.

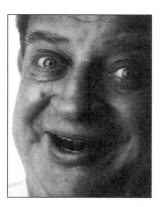

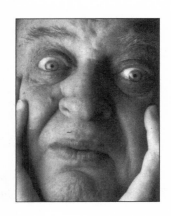

My psychiatrist told me I'm going crazy.
I told him, "I'd like a second opinion."
He said, "All right, you're ugly, too."

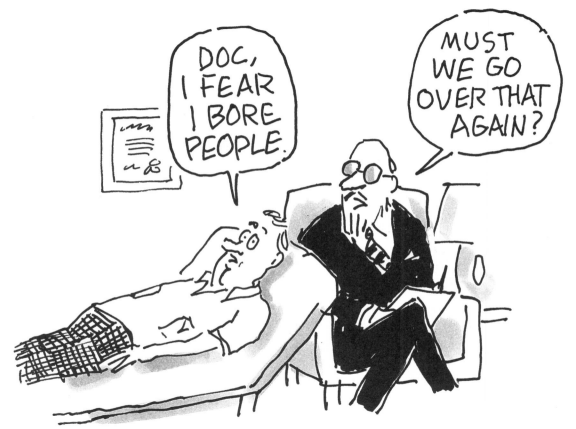

141

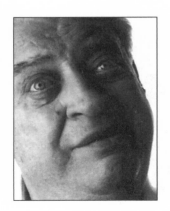

What a childhood I had. My parents sent me to a child psychiatrist. The kid didn't help me at all.

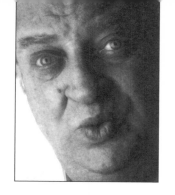

My psychiatrist told me
my wife and I should have sex every night....
Now we'll never see each other.

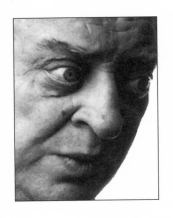

I told my psychiatrist I have suicidal tendencies.... He told me from now on I have to pay in advance.

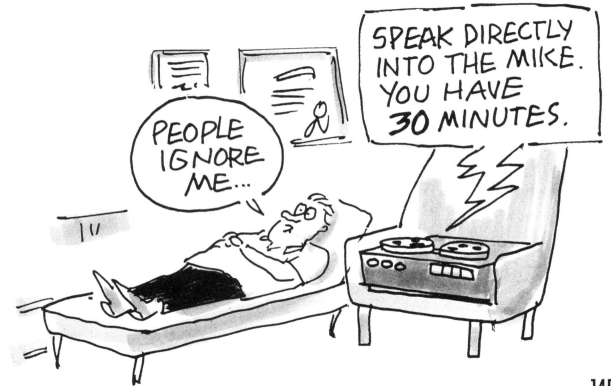

145

I told my doctor, "When I look
in the mirror, I wanna throw up.
What's wrong with me?"
He said, "I don't know,
but your eyesight's perfect."

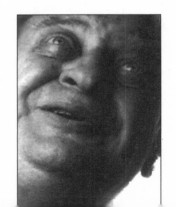

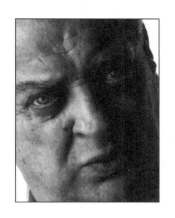

My doctor told me to run five miles a day
for two weeks.... I called him up. I said,
"Hey, Doc, I'm seventy miles from my house."

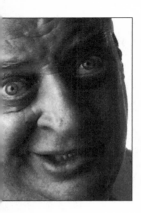

I told my doctor, "I think my wife has V.D."
He gave *himself* a shot of penicillin.

And my dentist. There's another one.
I told him to put in a new tooth
to match my other teeth....
He put in a tooth with four cavities.

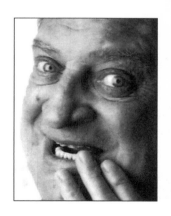

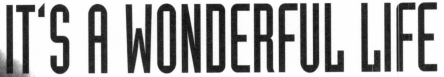

# IT'S A WONDERFUL LIFE

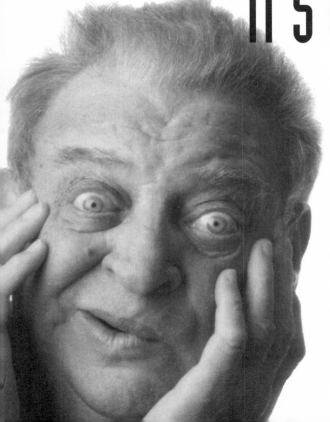

I tell ya, all I meet is wise guys. A travel agent told me I could spend six nights in Puerto Rico. No days, just nights. I said to him, "What will I do with myself days?" He said, "Do whatever you want, just keep out of Puerto Rico."

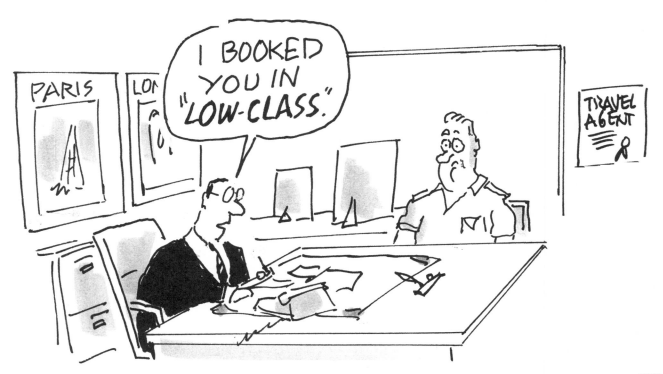

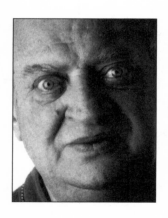

I tell ya, I don't get no respect.... American Airlines thanked me for flying United.

I flew no-frills.... I finished eating and had to do the dishes.

My last flight was a beauty....
The pilot made a left turn...
he put his hand out.

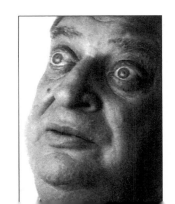

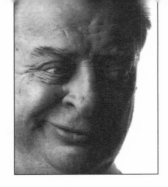

I went to buy a suit.
I told the salesman I wanna
see something cheap....
He told me to look in the mirror.

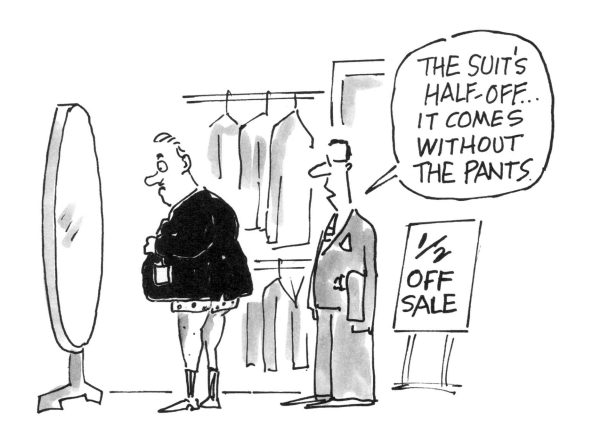

155

I don't get no respect from anyone.
I called Suicide Prevention....
They tried to talk me into it.

I called Gamblers Anonymous....
They gave me two-to-one odds
I wouldn't make it.

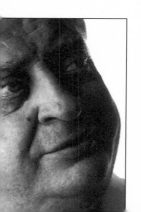

I met the Surgeon General,
he offered me a cigarette.

My bank told me they'll give me
a free gift if I close my account.

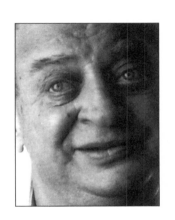

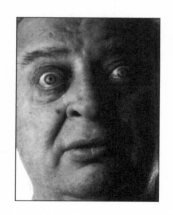

Yesterday was a beauty. I put on
my shirt and a button fell off....
I picked up my briefcase,
the handle fell off.... I'm afraid
to go to the bathroom.

So that's it, folks. I hope you liked the book. And if you didn't like it, let me know.... I'll do it over again.

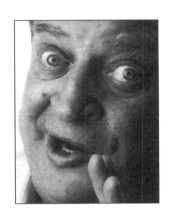

## ABOUT THE AUTHOR

RODNEY DANGERFIELD is known to millions for his critically acclaimed performances in comedies such as *Caddyshack*, *Easy Money,* and *Back to School* and dramas such as *Natural Born Killers.* A multimedia phenomenon, Dangerfield won a Grammy Award for his album *No Respect*, garnered accolades for his MTV video *Rockin' Rodney,* and has established himself as pitchman extraordinaire in commercials seen by audiences numbering in the billions. He has appeared on *The Tonight Show* seventy times and received the Creative Achievement Award for 1995 from the 9th Annual American Comedy Awards.

At the age of twenty-eight, Dangerfield actually quit show business, though at the time his profile was so low, he was the only one who knew it. Today, even at the summit of his profession, he offers cautionary advice to those who'd follow in his footsteps. As he told the Harvard College graduating class, "It's tough out there, don't go. Stay with your parents. Let them worry about it."

## ABOUT THE ILLUSTRATORS

BILL and ERIC TEITELBAUM are creators of the nationally syndicated business cartoon *Bottom Liners,* distributed by Tribune Media Services. Eric's cartoons also appear in *Forbes* and *The New Yorker*. Brother Bill doubles as an award-winning graphic designer.